I0434471

Table of Contents

Introduction to mirror-imaging:

Planning to do an activity requires you to create an image of what you want to do. This is how you go about your activities and the usual way you map out your day. But, what you may not suspect is that another part of the brain is watching you create this plan at the same time you are.

They are mirror cells, and they are more aware of what you need to do, to get things done than you might be.

There are thousands of them, and you wouldn't suspect that they could assist you the way they do, but they can, and they do this hundreds of times a day.

They pick up on your thoughts, of what you say, and how you look at a motor part of the body, so they can prepare you for this activity. And they do this by seeing what you see, and then absorbing the image.

This is when they get to work to absorb the peripheral image that you see of the front part of your body, that includes the tops of the shoulders, front of the arms and hands, and the lower part of the body that includes the feet. They see the same image you see of these motor parts and start to sort through it, to be sure that it looks like the last image you absorbed.

Some of the things they check to be sure you can identify with the image, are if you are able to use certain features, such as detecting feelings in the joints and the muscles to be sure you know how the joints are positioned, and if you are holding the arms the right way. For the hands, they expect you to recognize certain features, such as the skin tone, lines on the fingers and knuckles and how you hold the wrist and hand as if these details are all that you need to know.

They expect you to check them often, and make sure that they look and feel the same way they did the last time you created the peripheral image.

The image must stay the same way, because one thing mirror cells aren't keen on, is if the image changes in some way. If you look at a side of the body, or hand that you don't recognize, or aren't able to notice how it is moving, or how the skin tone matches the other hand, then, this makes the image harder to absorb.

Mirror cells won't absorb this image, because they need one that matches what is stored in the permanent memory in the brain. This image tells them how the peripheral image should look, such as how you hold the arms, and how you are supposed to imagine the shoulders look at a certain angle.

All of this is so you will be able to get motor functions and a memory back of how to perform the task, but also to allow you to think through the task and know how to visualize how the motor parts look while you are using it for an activity.

The cells look for certain types of behavior that signal that you know you are aware of the image, such as planning to look at the motor parts in the mirror and recognizing how the motor parts of the body should look when you look at them from a peripheral image angle.

These actions, of needing to look at the motor parts, believing that they belong to you, are called intentions, or purposeful gestures, that signal that you can have control of these motor parts of the body.

These intentions also tell the mirror cells that you know that you need to absorb the motor parts of the body and that you know that both sides of the body need to look the same way. At least this is what these actions project to the mirror cells.

Absorbing images improves your chances for attracting mirror cells to your image, and returns motor functions, and skills, such as planning, recognition, and perception that restore you to a level of peripheral imaging that will increase your productivity and allow you to be more aware of how you move and when you move.

If you've had a stroke or brain injury, the ability to absorb these images is affected, because the images look different now, on both sides of the body. Muscle movement can be difficult because the brain isn't receiving the messages it needs for the kind of activity you want to do. Trying to recall the image you just looked at is hard because you aren't using these places in the brain that you need to process an image. Imaging can bring back these motor functions by supplying the brain with the visual image you need of how a motor part looks to you, and allow you feel in charge of these tasks again.

Chapter 1: The mirror cell image

Mirror cells absorb three kinds of peripheral images: one of the upper body, which includes the shoulders, arms, and hands, the shoulders in the mirror, and the legs and feet.

Mirror cells absorb your image two ways: by you recognizing the traits of the motor part, such as the shape of the shoulders, and arms, and the other way is by showing the intent of needing to use the motor part and having a plan to use the motor part.

Intent or a purposeful gesture can be shown a few ways, such as having a plan to look at the motor part of the body or trying to determine is the muscles in the shoulder work the same way on each side of the shoulder. Intent can be a simple gesture too, such as needing to look at the shoulders a certain way in the mirror.

A gesture, of needing to look at the shoulders in the mirror, is enough to tell the mirror cells that you have a purpose for looking at the shoulders, and that you believe that you need to see both shoulders at the same time.

The cells recognize this gesture and see it as a sign that you are in control of the need to look at the image and deliver it to the brain. This approach works when you have a brain injury too and is a way to attract mirror cells when the image that you see is less than perfect in the mirror.

This intent approach when looking at a partial peripheral image in the mirror, tells you what mirror cells are looking for in the image you see in the mirror. This would be if you were planning an activity, knew that you had to look at the image, or were attempting to compare how the two shoulders look.

The intent method can be used to overcome the visual symptoms that you have if you are still recovering from a stroke, such as having blurry vision that you see when you look in the mirror. This is usually a blurry shoulder or blotchy shoulder if you have been to therapy but are still having trouble with this image.

Absorbing a partial image:

Though the image will start to improve on its own when you look in the mirror, within a few weeks, and then you will feel that you are gaining control, you don't want to wait this long to try to show that you need to look at the image. The longer you wait the more the brain heals, without having the most ability to function back. The motor neurons won't be able to repair the places in the brain that still need to heal if they don't receive activity in the form of visual images.

The brain only wants to see mirror images for anything that has to do with motor images. So, if you aren't able to see all of the images, such as the shoulder, you need to find another way to deliver the image to the brain, other than visual, and so the intent approach works to deliver images to the brain of how you think about the motor parts, and also your plans or purposeful gestures about what you are going to do with the images. This can be to look at the image, study certain parts of the motor image, such as the muscles around the shoulders, or imagine that the motor parts work. All of these are planned activities with a purpose, and this is the kind of thinking that mirror cells want to see.

This can be shown by forming a plan of needing to look in the mirror or having a need to look at an image or deciding that you want to compare the two shoulder muscles.

Any of these actions indicate to mirror cells that you need to look at the image, and that you know that you need to include it in the peripheral image of the upper body.

Another form of intent is to pretend that one side of the body works as well as the other one. This is to show that you want to include this side of the body in the image.

There is another method of intent if you can't see the image, that will allow you to place your eyes on the right location of the shoulder joints in the mirror and show mirror cells that you do know where the right place is to put your eyes. This method uses an alternative background to focus your eyes on as you try to lift them to a shoulder. A patterned shirt works for you to rest your eyes on the designs of the stomach, and then be able to focus them on what you see in the shoulder.

The shirt:

The shirt acts like resting place, on the way up to the shoulders, and acts as a navigation tool too, to bring yourself up to the affected shoulder and leave your eyes in this place for two seconds.

The focus becomes the shirt, rather than trying to sort out where to place your eyes on the blurry or blotchy image, so you can get them on the right location, and feel as if you have looked at the shoulder image on your own. This is a way to see the peripheral image of the shoulders, with the least amount of sorting out of the image as possible.

This short visit to the mirror, with the placement of the eyes on the right location of the shoulders, is enough to have mirror cells absorb some of the image and return some of the motor functions have the skills you need to plan out your visual image.

Mirror cells will react the same way they always do, but you may not realize that you are getting the motor functions back, because you aren't able to retain all the images.

As the image becomes clearer, and you will be able to focus more on the task, you will be more aware of improved concentration, focus, and levels of planning that go along with the returned motor functions and skills.

You will place your eyes on the middle of the shirt, to get your bearings, and then when you are ready, bring your eyes up to the middle of the shirt-sleeve, over where you know the round part of the shoulder is located. This allows you to capture the image of where the round shoulder joint is located, in the middle of the shirt sleeve, and then leave the mirror.

This shortens your stay in front of the mirror to a few seconds, rather than linger over the image for longer than you need to. This gets your image done and leaves you with time to rest before you return to the mirror again for another image.

This short exercise of needing to place your eyes on the affected shoulder is enough time to be able to create activity in the brain allows the mirror cells to absorb some of the image.

The design:

Wear a shirt with a design pattern that covers the whole shirt, such as leaves, bells or cityscapes, that allows you to see the pattern at once. This allows you to find a design quickly, because there are so many, and you simply need to look at a canvas of the shirt, to be able to pick out a few. This makes finding a place to put your eyes easier, and less work.

The shirt should have a light-colored pattern such as celery green, mocha, copper, expresso, light-blue, beige and light gray works great to relax the eyes and allow you to pick out the design easily.

The designs on the shirt give you something more tangible to look at, rather than a solid colored shirt, which causes the background to blend and makes it harder for you to decipher where you are located on the shirt.

The shirt acts as a reminder of your past too, of the person you were before the injury, and gives you an uplifting feeling, of hope that you will get back to that person.

Make sure this shirt is a short-sleeved shirt, and that it fits snuggly or tightly, so you can make out the outline of the round part of the shoulders more easily in the mirror.

After this, you are ready to proceed to the mirror and work on bringing your eyes up to the shirt-sleeve on your own.

Exercise 1.0: How to bring the eyes up to the affected shirt-sleeve (use for 2x day)

1. Wear your patterned shirt
2. Stand in front of the mirror
3. Focus your eyes on the stomach region of the shirt for several seconds
4. This is how much space you need to rest your eyes – four to six designs.
5. Rest the eyes on the designs of the stomach for 2 minutes
6. When ready, try to bring eyes up to the middle design on the shirt sleeve on the affected shoulder. This is the design directly over the round shoulder joint beneath the sleeve.
7. Keep them here for two seconds.
8. Rest for up to 2 hours. Then try the exercise again.

The stomach serves as a safe-haven to place your eyes, but measuring space can be difficult, so you want to try to count out how many designs you have in the middle of the shirt within the clear portion of the shirt. This will tell you how much width you have in the stomach region and know that the number of designs in this space will always stay the same.

You can plan to place your eyes on these designs each time you go to the mirror and know that your eyes are safe. This will not change. And, so you can then plan to bring your eyes up to the shirt sleeve gradually, by focusing on how many designs you have in the shirt sleeve region, and then placing your eyes there.

The Pattern for placing eyes on shirt-sleeve:

1. Keep eyes on the stomach for a minute
2. Look up at the shirt-sleeve briefly
3. Notice where the clear design is located on the sleeve
4. Pick the middle design
5. When ready bring eyes up to this clear design

Finding a clear design in the middle of the shirt-sleeve ahead of time is a way of securing where you need to place your eyes before you move them. This is also a way to show that you know where the round part of the shirt-sleeve is located, such as over the sleeve, and a way to show the brain that you know where you need to place your eyes.

If you were to look in the mirror at the sleeves, it would be over the round part of the shirt-sleeves because this is the place that you are used to looking at the round part of the shirt-sleeves. This is where you have always placed your eyes and should keep placing your eyes, to show that you are looking at both shoulders in the mirror. This is also how you looked at the shoulders in the mirror in the past, and so there is a memory of you doing this on file in the brain.

Practice: bringing the eyes up to the shirt-sleeve

1. Wear your patterned shirt
2. Stand in front of the mirror
3. Focus your eyes on the stomach region of the shirt first
4. Find four to six designs that you can see clearly and keep your eyes on this set of details.
5. This is how much space you can use, to rest your eyes – four to six designs.
6. When ready, try to bring eyes up to the middle design of the affected shirt sleeve. This is the one directly over the round shoulder joint.
7. Keep your eyes here for 2 seconds.
8. Take a rest for up to 2 hours. Then try the exercise again.

Treat the exercise like a task, one that you need to do, but will only last a few seconds, and then you can rest. So, the plan is to go to the mirror, place your eyes on the stomach, leave them there for a few seconds, and then bring them back to the stomach. Then leave the mirror.

Rest periods:

During the first four weeks of looking in the mirror, you will need to rest for up to two hours at a time. This allows the image to process in the brain, the way it usually would, and starts to rebuild a pattern that the brain is used to doing, which is absorbing the images on its own.

Thresholds:

This is when you may start to notice some physical symptoms crop up when you are in front of the mirror that let you know that you have reached the threshold of absorption. The threshold is for the brain as well, to let you know that it can't absorb any more of the image than it already has, and so you want to find a place to sit. This will allow you to finish processing the image and let you rest at the same time.

Symptoms include dizziness, sudden loss of focus, and a feeling of strain in the eyes. These are all signs that you need to sit down and take a rest.

Checkpoint: Do this shirt exercise 2x a day for 1 – 3 weeks. Notice when the image starts to improve but be careful not to go over the two-second threshold, to be sure that you stay within the absorption levels.

Chapter 2: Identify with the shoulder

If you are experiencing a lack of identity of the affected shoulder, such as forgetting how it works, or have a section that you can't see, or know how the muscles feel, then you'll have to attract mirror cells another way, by pointing out how the shoulders look on the outside.

Though you may not be able to absorb the whole image, you will be able to absorb a partial image, if you deliver the same train of thought as you did before, when studying how the shoulders look.

To do this, you will have to use an obvious gesture, such as pulling back the shirtsleeves, and looking at how the muscles of the shoulder are shaped, and how they flex. This is to get the brain to notice that you are looking at two identical images.

This intentional gesture of wanting to look at both bare shoulders tells the mirror cells that you have a purpose for looking at the shoulders, and that you feel that both shoulders look the same.

The two tasks in this exercise are to look at the bare shoulders, which will bring the brain back to the basics of when you first looked at the shoulders and give you a way to show the brain that you do know how the shoulders work. And the other task is to question why one shoulder doesn't work as well as the other one. This questioning approach allows you to be able to give a reason as to why you think the two shoulders are the same and point out that there are too many similarities for the affected shoulder not to work.

These intent gestures will attract mirror cells to your image.

This is your platform, to show the brain that you are familiar with the shoulders on a basic level, and you can point out the similarities if you need to, and make these images look more similar than they do.

Exercise 2.0: Notice that the two bare shoulders look the same (use for 2x day)

1. Stand in front of the mirror
2. Look at the healthy shoulder first, pull back the shirtsleeve, and study the bare-skinned shoulder.
3. Then, look over at the affected shoulder, and pull back this sleeve, and study this bare-skinned shoulder.
4. Notice how this round muscle of the shoulder looks.
5. Use a verbal command that says, "This shoulder looks the same as the healthy one."

Inspecting the shoulders, such noticing how the muscles look around the joint, is a way to try to convince the mirror cells that you agree that the muscles and joints work the same way.

So, if you are observing the round parts of the shoulders in the mirror, and saying to yourself, that "these two shoulders look the same," then the mirror cells will see this as a sign that you want to use these bare shoulders for an activity.

There will be less eye strain, and less resistance when you look in the mirror at the shoulders this way, because the brain does not associate looking at bare shoulders, with that of preparing for an activity with the arms, as much as when you are looking directly at the shoulders in the shirt in the mirror.

But it is possible to have mirror cells absorb this perfect image of the bare shoulder, because you are looking at two identical images of the shoulders, and you are examining them, to determine if they can be used in an activity the same way.

Exercise 2.1: Study the bare shoulder muscles in the mirror (use for 2x day)

1. Stand in the mirror in your patterned shirt

2. Pull back the short sleeve of the healthy shoulder

3. Pull back the short sleeve of the affected shoulder

4. Say, "These two shoulders look alike."

5. Study how the round muscles of the shoulder look

6. Notice that the affected shoulder muscles are shaped the same way

7. Say "It looks like these two shoulders work the same way."

8. Notice the skin color, and the way the clavicle meets the shoulder

9. Say, "I believe these two shoulders can work the same way."

10. Take a rest for two hours.

Say that "they must be made the same way," tells the brain that you can't find evidence that the shoulders are different, and this begins to show the brain that you are nearly convinced that these two shoulders work the same way and look the same way.

Another piece of evidence, that you find is that when you look at the bare shoulders, as you study them in the mirror: "this shoulder looks just like the other one," almost as an observation, of seeing that the affected shoulder does look the same. This surprised tone also points out your disbelief that the affected shoulder could look any different, and so you are wondering what all the fuss is about.

You are the investigator in this case and the one in charge of trying to find similarities with how the shoulders look.

The brain is used to seeing the outline of the shoulders with your patterned shirt on, in preparation for activity, but it will accept this less obvious image of you looking at the bare-skinned shoulders, as a way for you to show that you believe that they can work.

The swing motion:

Another obvious gesture to show how the shoulders are made the same way is to swing the shoulders in place for a few seconds in front of the mirror and observe how the round joints of the shoulders feel.

The swing motion:

1. Keep arms bent, and loose so they swing on the shoulder joint
2. Keep hands loose or in a loose fist

This is the position of the arms that you use when you want to swing them back, and forth, to feel how the muscles over the shoulder joint feel, and to try to make sure you are aligning the shoulders the right way.

This is a way for you to show how similar the shoulders are in the mirror image, at least on the outside, because when you swing the arms, both shoulder joints appear to look the same – smooth, round, similar shape.

This obvious gesture of swinging the arms in place is another obvious gesture to let the mirror cells know that you can move the arms the same way, and this shows that they are similar. The fact that you see a round shoulder joint on both arms, creates another duel image and lets the brain know that these two shoulders have the same joints.

Exercise 2.2: Study the shoulders in swing motion (use for 2x day)

1. Stand in front of the mirror with the pattern shirt on

2. Be up close to the mirror

3. Pull back the healthy shoulder shirtsleeve

4. Study the muscles on the bare-skinned shoulder

5. Pull back the affected shoulder shirtsleeve

6. Study the muscles on the bare-skinned shoulder

7. Begin to swing the arms slightly

8. Notice the shape of the shoulders

9. Keep eyes on the shoulders for a few more seconds

10. Leave the mirror to rest.

This similarity of how the two shoulder joints look, makes you feel as if you can use both these shoulders the same way, and that you believe they both work the same way.

This investigative approach toward swinging the shoulders and then trying to detect if both have the tension at the front of the shoulders also shows that you believe that the tension exists in both shoulders (internal image), but that you are searching for it on the affected shoulder, because it is not as obvious on this shoulder.

Checkpoint: Work on these exercises 2x day for three weeks. As you do the exercises you may start to become familiar with having to include the affected shoulder in the activity. This is the intent, to try to show that you want to include the affected side in your peripheral image of the shoulders, but that you are still working on identifying with a few traits.

Chapter 3: Past and present images

Past images can be used to imagine that you can use the affected shoulder, but also to remind you of how you used to move the shoulder. This is also an internal image, because you are planning to picture an image of the shoulder, and any time you plan an activity with the shoulder it shows purpose and the ability to show that you want to bring back the image.

The memory of how the affected shoulder worked in the past, allows you to wonder how the muscles on the affected shoulder work, so you can try to formulate how you would be able to do this on your own.

Your intention for using the image is to try to discover how you moved your shoulder in the past when you stood in front of the mirror. This start with having to remember a time when you were in front of the mirror. At this time, you looked at the shoulders, and then you noticed that you were able to move the shoulder. You were able to move it well and know why you were moving it this way.

Past images are also internal images, which are images that you create of how the inside of the shoulder works as best you can. To imagine how the inside of the shoulder works, is still the same process if it is a past image or present image, and so the mirror cells will recognize this effort as one that is the same as how you used to create the internal image.

This is also identity because you are trying to imagine that the muscles work on both shoulders. You will examine how the muscles look in the mirror, for both shoulders, and then tell yourself that the ones on the affected shoulder look the same as the ones on the healthy shoulder.

If you imagine that the shoulder works a certain way, or that you want it to work a certain way, then you are wishing that it would work like the healthier one. This is a form of comparison and an attempt to try and recognize how the muscles and the bones and tendons work on the affected side, and a form of wondering how the two shoulders work.

Example 3.0: Create a past memory of the shoulder

1. Stand in front of the mirror
2. Focus on the round shoulders in the short-sleeved pattern shirt
3. Pull back the shirt-sleeves
4. Notice how the muscles look on the healthy shoulder
5. Then look at the muscles on the affected shoulder
6. Think back to a time when you could use these affected shoulder muscles
7. Imagine that you can move the shoulder and arm the same way.
8. Form an image in your mind of when you moved the shoulder in the past.
9. Hold onto the image for a few seconds
10. Take a rest.

In this image, you were studying how the muscles on the affected shoulder, look and then imagining that you are the person you used to be, with two working shoulders.

Now, as you stare at the muscles, and how they look on the affected shoulder in the mirror, you picture this shoulder suddenly move, just briefly, for a few seconds, as if by magic it just moved, in a wispy dream, and then went back to being in place again. This is a past image, of imagining that the shoulder moved, for a second, as you used to move it, and then it returned to looking as it does in the mirror.

Example 3.1: The wispy dream past image

1. Stand in front of the mirror in the patterned shirt

2. Look at the shoulders in the shirt

3. Pull back the shirt sleeve on the healthy shoulder to study the muscles

4. Pull back the shirt sleeve on the affected shoulder to study the muscles

5. Think of how well the muscles work on healthy shoulder

6. Study how the affected bare shoulder muscles look in the mirror.

7. Think back to when you could move the bare shoulder in the mirror

8. Now imagine that you can move this shoulder briefly, for a few seconds.

9. Then return to the shoulder image you see in the mirror.

10. Take a rest.

So, with this image, you decide for a few brief seconds, that you want to be like the person you used to be when you could picture yourself using the bare shoulder in the mirror. For a few seconds, your shoulder could work, and you forgot that you have a problem trying to decide how you would use it. Now, for a few seconds, you are that person again, who is capable and can look in the mirror, and know how the shoulder looks and feels. You are this person again, and you can imagine that this shoulder works when you need it to. This is a purposeful gesture, and a visual image of the shoulder, which will provide the activity to the brain, and heal places that need repairs. These wispy past images, are also motor images to the brain and will attract mirror cells to your image, attempting to return motor functions to you, as well as skills for evaluating the image and how it looks compared to how the healthy one looks.

Exercise 3.2: Think back to when you could use the shoulder (use for 2x day)

1. Stand in front of the mirror, in patterned shirt

2. Pull back the shirtsleeves

3. Study the bare shoulder on the healthy side

4. Study the bare shoulder on the affected side

5. Look at the muscles on the bare shoulder of the affected side

6. Think back to when you could use the bare shoulder and studied it in the mirror.

7. Imagine you are this person

8. Feel as capable as this person

9. And that moving the shoulder is an afterthought

10. You simply move it if you want to.

11. Take a rest.

The shoulder may or may not move, in this example, depending on how well you are able to absorb the image and attract mirror cells to your image. But, the mirror cells will be attracted to the image, in some way so the image will be partially absorbed, and you will get back some motor functions to this side of the body.

When you get back the motor functions, you are then able to think through movements, plan, and focus on how to move the arm, and know why you are supposed to compare the two shoulders and arms. You may be aware that these functions returned if you are able to keep them in your memory, otherwise, you will just feel as if you can concentrate more and stay focused in the mirror.

Past Images show recognition:

Trying to get this image of the muscles to look more like the one that you see on the healthy shoulder, is a form of showing that you want to use this affected shoulder again but are still working on getting this image to look like the one you have on your healthy side. You created the internal image, even though you had one that looked faded, and was missing a lot of the thought processes, such as identity, and visual imaging that you usually create.

Taking the initiative to create an internal image of the shoulder, is another form of getting back to what you would normally do if you were trying to think of how the shoulder works. This is an image that you will need to create when you begin to use the peripheral image of the upper body on your own.

This allows the mirror cells to take an interest in the image you create, first, because of the partial image you are trying to form, that resembles one that you created in the past. The thought that you are trying to picture yourself as being more like the past, and the idea that you imagine your shoulder can work as well as the healthy one, allow mirror cells to believe that you can use the shoulder almost as much as the healthy one, and they will absorb some of the image.

Mirror cells react to any thoughts you have of wanting to use a motor part of the body, even if it is an image of the past. This is still a thought, or wonder that you have about the image, and how the muscles work, and so this is a sign that you are trying to show that you are taking charge of the shoulder.

Though this image only appears for a short time, you are still exercising the brain, and providing it with activity.

Present images:

For this type of exercise, you'll examine the shoulders, and disclaim the notion that the affected shoulder isn't working as well as the healthy side. Studying the shoulders this way, makes you think that the affected shoulder should work and that it must work, based on the idea that the muscles seem to look the same on the healthy side, and therefore, they must work the same way.

Exercise 3.3: Study how the shoulders look presently (Use for 2x day)

1. Look in the mirror at the healthy shoulder
2. Study the bare-skinned image of the healthy shoulder and affected one
3. Notice how the muscles are shaped on each one
4. Imagine that you know how these muscles work
5. Imagine that you can move the affected shoulder
6. Say "these muscles look the same, I must be able to use this shoulder."
7. Study how the muscles look on the healthy shoulder and then the affected one.
8. Wait to see if mirror cells react
9. Move one shoulder forward, and the other one back
10. Imagine that you can use them the same way
11. Spend three minutes doing this.
12. Notice if the image returns of you just knowing how the shoulder works suddenly

Studying the bare shoulders this way, after an injury to the brain takes longer, and the mirror cells need to be convinced for a few minutes before they decide to absorb some of your image.

When the memory returns, it will arrive in the form of suddenly having knowledge of how to move the shoulder, and that you are noticing how the shoulders look in the mirror. It will seem as if you have just slipped back into your old way of thinking and that you are able to feel that you recognize how the how you used to look at them in the shirt, and suddenly know how the shoulder is made and how it works.

As if someone has waved a magic wand and allowed you to return to yourself for just a short time, you are able to see how everything works and feel as if the shoulder works fine. And wondering what all the fuss is about.

Then, as quickly as this ability surfaces, it goes away. As if you never had it back, and you are left with the shoulder that you hardly recognize again.

This takes longer if you've had a brain injury, and so you need to look at the shoulders for about three minutes. But, the mirror cells can respond if you study the shoulders long enough and imagine that the shoulder muscles work again.

Exercise 3.4: Study how the shoulders look presently (Use for 2x day)

1. Look in the mirror at the healthy shoulder
2. Study the bare-skinned image of the healthy shoulder and affected one
3. Notice how the muscles are shaped on each one
4. Imagine that you know how these muscles work
5. Imagine that you can move the affected shoulder
6. Say "these muscles look the same, I must be able to use this shoulder."
7. Study how the muscles look on the healthy shoulder and then the affected one.
8. Wait to see if mirror cells react

9. Move one shoulder forward, and the other one back

10. Imagine that you can use them the same way

11. Spend three minutes doing this.

12. Notice if the image returns of you just knowing how the shoulder works suddenly

Exercise 3.5: Study the shoulders to bring back movement (use for 2x day)

1. Stand in front of the mirror in the patterned shirt

2. Study how the shoulders look in the patterned shirt

3. Do this for several seconds

4. Turn down the shirt-sleeve on both shoulders

5. Say "this shoulder looks and feels the same way as the healthy shoulder."

6. Bring shirt-sleeves up, and study how they look

7. Look from shirt-sleeve to shirt-sleeve as if both shoulders are the same

8. Now look directly at the affected shoulder and count to ten or twenty on this shoulder

9. Inspect how the shoulder looks in the shirt.

10. Leave the mirror and rest.

So, here a lot of inspection went on over a period of nearly three minutes, looking back and forth from one shoulder to the other one. You always want to pretend that the affected shoulder looks and works as well as the other shoulder, because this is what you wish, and mirror cells will see this as a means, to a task.

Exercise 3.6: Study the affected shoulder (2x day)

1. Say, "I plan to study the shoulders to bring back motion."

2. Approach the mirror in your shirt.

3. Study the two shoulders in the short-sleeved patterned shirt

4. Look at how the round shoulder joint looks in the affected shirt sleeve

5. Study the round joint outline.

6. Then the affected side.

7. Say, "This side works as well as the healthy side."

8. Keep studying the affected shoulder, by pulling back the shirt-sleeve and then looking at the outline of the shirt.

9. Look back at the healthy shoulder in the shirt-sleeve

10. Say "I need this shoulder to work as well as the healthy shoulder works."

11. Then look back at the affected shoulder

12. Say, "I need this shoulder to work as well as the other shoulder."

13. A few more seconds, and then you should feel that you suddenly know how to use this affected shoulder on your own. (Motion memory).

14. Rest for an hour.

You should be looking at the affected shoulder when you say that you "want the affected shoulder to work as well as the healthy one." This is a wish you have for the affected shoulder to work as well as the healthy one, and when you wish for something to do with the motor parts of the body, this too is considered a planned activity with the motor parts and attracts mirror cells.

Example 3.7: Picture the affected shoulder working for motion

1. Stand in front of the mirror.

2. Study the healthy shoulder in the patterned shirt-sleeve

3. Pull back the sleeve to see the bare skin of the shoulder

4. Do the same on the other side

5. Then study how the affected shoulder looks

6. Say "this shoulder should work the same way as the other one."

7. Picture the muscles of the affected shoulder working.

8. Without moving the shoulder picture being able to move this shoulder on your own

9. Imagine that you know how to move the affected shoulder

10. Pull back the shirtsleeve on the affected shoulder

11. Keep imaging that this shoulder can work

12. Do this for about a minute

13. You should suddenly realize how to move the shoulder and arm.

This is the same idea as if you used a present image, of studying how the shoulder looked in the bare-skinned shoulders and then imagining that the shoulders work the same way and that you believe that the affected shoulder is the same as the healthy one. As you study the affected shoulder for several minutes and also think that you want the shoulder to work, and that it should work this is the same kind of thinking that you would normally do, to try to get the shoulder to work, inspecting it, and then studying how it works, along with how it works on the inside of the shoulder.

Say you have a plan:

Voice prompts work because they are a way to send a message to the brain that you are working with motor parts, other than trying to think of the image. Trying to think of the image takes a lot of work, because you need to picture yourself at the location for the image, and then picture what you want to do for the image, but prompts get the attention of mirror images, because you are thinking of the motor part of the body.

Example 3.8: say you have a plan

1. Before you get to the mirror, say, "I plan to inspect the shoulders in the mirror."

2. Approach the mirror in the patterned shirt

3. Study how the shoulders look in the patterned shirt

This plan shows that you want to inspect the shoulders in the mirror and that you approached the mirror and followed through with the plan.

Make a schedule:

This gets mirror cells attention because you are thinking of an activity you plan to do with motor parts of the body. As you think through which activities you plan, the mirror cells can deliver some motor functions, if you are able to identify with the motor parts the way you did before.

Making a schedule also allows you to track your progress, as you go along in the weeks.

Example of a schedule:

1. In the morning – stand in front of the mirror for two seconds 2x day

2. Keep track of threshold

3. Rest for an hour

4. At lunch – try the foot exercise 1x day

5. Keep track of threshold

6. Rest for an hour

7. At dinner – stand in front of the mirror for two seconds

8. Keep track of threshold

9. Rest for an hour.

In this schedule, you are planning to look in the mirror in the morning, and at dinner, but only look at the shoulders for three seconds each in the morning. This means that after you have looked at your shoulders for three seconds, you are done with this task, and can leave the mirror to rest for up to two hours.

Morning plan for 6 A.M.:

Study the shoulders in the mirror in the morning – two seconds, for each shoulder

1. Say "I have a plan to look at my shoulders in the mirror."
2. Approach mirror in the shirt.
3. Look at the shirt-sleeve of the healthy shoulder two seconds
4. Look at the shirt-sleeve of the affected shoulder two seconds
5. Leave the mirror and rest.

This is your morning plan, for which you have added the "have a plan," prompt, to your schedule, so you remember to think of your plan, as you approach the mirror.

So, the plan for 6 A.M. is to look in the mirror at the healthy shoulder for two seconds, and then at the affected shoulder for two seconds. Then leave the mirror.

Trace images:

If you are recovering from a stroke, then trace images may appear in your thoughts as you recover. They are wispy images of memories that you have of looking in the mirror, such as seeing a portion of the patterned shirt, in the stomach region or the shirt sleeves.

This is not a sign that anything is wrong, but rather, that the brain is trying to restore memories of how you look in the mirror. And soon as they appear they are gone, and then you are left with only the present memories of what you see in front of you.

Checkpoint: Work on these exercises for about two weeks, 2x day. Among the exercises, try to picture past images of the shoulders, for two seconds. Then try to create the return of the mirror cell memory, by studying the affected shoulder in the mirror for three minutes.

Chapter 4: Glimpse the shoulders

Glimpsing is a way to practice trying to detect feelings in the shoulders and try to associate one shoulder to the other. Trying to imagine that you can see an internal image of the shoulder, and one that is the same as the other one, is a way to bring you closer to regaining this image. If you can associate one shoulder with the other one and start to glimpse more often at the affected shoulder, then you weave in the behavior that you had before the injury.

This allows you to start to include the affected shoulder in the peripheral image and to begin to treat the shoulder as if it works the same way as the healthy shoulder.

Steps: for glimpsing

1. Stand in front of the mirror
2. Notice how you look in the shirt-sleeves
3. Notice the details of the sleeve, the edging of the sleeve
4. Notice how the upper arms look
5. Step away from the mirror
6. Try to remember how you look in the shirt-sleeve
7. Glimpse down at the two shoulders
8. Try to detect the nudging feeling in front of the healthy shoulder
9. Then try to determine if it there on the affected one
10. Leave the mirror and rest

Practice studying how you look in the patterned shirt, and then turn away from the mirror and try to remember how you looked in the shirt. Try to remember details of the boatneck on the shirt (if you have one), and the thick green seam on the shirt-sleeve (or another kind of sleeve) and try to picture how the front of the arms look, and the skin tone. Do this for a few seconds at a time.

Exercise 4.1: Study how you look in the mirror and then try to remember the details of the shirt (use for 2x)

1. Stand in front of the mirror
2. Notice how you look in the shirt-sleeves
3. Notice the details of the sleeve, the edging of the sleeve
4. Notice how the upper arms look
5. Turn away from the mirror
6. Try to remember how you looked in the shirt
7. Try to picture the details of the neckline, and how the upper arms look
8. Take a rest.

This is also an identity exercise to see if you can remember the details of the shirt in the chest region. This is one of the places that you will have to include in your peripheral image, when you stand at the sink or try to reach for something.

Exercise 4.2: Study how you look in the mirror and then look down at the shoulders (use for 2x a day)

1. Stand in front of the mirror
2. Notice how you look in the shirt-sleeves
3. Notice the details of the sleeve, the edging of the sleeve
4. Notice how the upper arms look

5. Turn away from the mirror

6. Try to remember how you looked in the shirt

7. Try to picture the details of the neckline, and how the upper arms look

8. Look down at the healthy arm

9. Study how it looks, from a top angle.

10. Look down at the affected arm

11. Study how it looks, from a top angle.

12. Do this for up to a minute.

13. Leave the mirror. Take a rest.

   Do this exercise, two more times.

   Stay on the shirt exercises in the mirror, for a while longer, if you need to, to study how the chest region in the patterned shirt looks, and the upper arms. Turn away from the mirror to try to remember how they look. Then move onto the next sections for glimpsing both sides.

   Exercise 4.3: Glimpse as you walk with voice prompts (use for 2x day)

1. Study how the shoulders look in the mirror

2. Study how the patterned shirt looks

3. Notice how the upper arms look

4. Turn away from the mirror

5. Try to imagine how you looked in the shirt in the mirror

6. Take a few steps away from the mirror

7. Look down at the healthy arm

8. Then, the affected arm

9. Pause

10. As you look at this arm, say, "this arm works the same way as the other arm."

11. Look up again, keep walking

12. Try to imagine the affected arm working as well as the healthy arm.

13. Look down at the arm again.

14. Take a rest.

If you feel that you have forgotten how to include the arm, pause and then look down at the patterned shirt, so you can get yourself back on track, before you start walking again. This is so you train the brain too, that you are trying to include the affected arm in the image,

The shoulder patch:

This is a colorful picture of a healthy shoulder, with a large white shoulder joint, ligaments and muscles that you can associate with how the other shoulder is made. Now you have a more colorful shoulder image, and a more robust one, for the affected side, and one that resembles how the internal image of the healthy shoulder looks.

This makes the two shoulder images appear more alike and seem as though you are aware of the internal image of the shoulder on this side of the body.

This should be a picture that you can follow as a guide for how the inside of the shoulder looks – white round cartilage joint, surrounded by ligaments, and smooth, contoured muscles shaped in a ball.

Choose a healthy, colorful photo of the anatomy of a shoulder, that has smooth contoured muscles, a round joint, like the shoulder, and represents what you think is a healthy version of your own shoulder.

This image gives you something tangible to work with, that is close to the internal image that you would normally create on the healthy side.

If the image is closer to the one you would normally create on the healthy side, then the mirror cells are more likely to react and absorb some of the image.

The paper image of the healthy shoulder creates a more realistic view of the shoulder and tells you that there is a working picture of a shoulder here. This idea that there is a shoulder here, will get you thinking of a working shoulder and have you comparing this shoulder to the healthy shoulder more often, which will start to send messages to the brain that this shoulder is just like your other one.

Tape this shoulder patch on the sleeve over the affected shoulder that you are having trouble seeing. Imagine that you need to glimpse down at it often, to be sure that it is working and that you know that you are supposed to be using this image as your shoulder.

Attach the picture to your affected shoulder

1. Cut out an anatomical version of your shoulder

2. Make sure you do this, to be sure it is your version of the shoulder.

3. Tape it on the shirt-sleeve of your affected shoulder

4. Look down at it often, as if you are checking it

5. Compare it to your healthy shoulder, as if it works.

This is now the shoulder that you take care of, that you think of, and look out for, and the one that you will imagine, when you think of creating the peripheral image of the shoulder.

If the picture gets wet or damaged in some way replace it with another copy of the same shoulder image. Keep spares stored in a clean plastic bag in case you lose this one and need to replace it.

Wear it when you are out, underneath your coat, so you know that it is there and that you can think of it whenever you want. Since it represents your shoulder, you should think of it as your real shoulder, and think of it as often as you do your healthy one.

What you are after:

This paper version of your healthy shoulder, with the perfectly arranged colorful picture of the joint, thick muscles and tendons, will quickly allow you to think of your affected shoulder more often, and you will check it, (or the paper image), by glimpsing, as you do the other side, to see if it moved, and to keep track of how it looks, and if it is still dry and in good condition.

As you compare the shoulders, you will start to look for similarities between how the healthy shoulder feels, and how the affected shoulder feels with the patch on. This can occur while you are out, wearing the patch, or when you are inside, doing the exercises, but you will start to feel something as you start to think of this patch shoulder more, such as control or focus, because both shoulder images receive the same motor memory.

You may start to picture the internal image of the healthy shoulder, for example, on the healthy side, and see a round thick muscle over the joint, and then suddenly feel that you notice the same thing on the affected side.

Exercise 4.4: Use the patch to detect a healthy internal image on the affected shoulder (use for 2x day)

1. Stand away from the mirror

2. Wear the patterned shirt

3. Place the patch on the affected shoulder

4. Glimpse down at the affected shoulder

5. Imagine that the inside of this shoulder has a white joint, and smooth muscles that appear in the picture.

6. Imagine that it has red tendons.

7. This is your internal image.

8. Now imagine that these parts are on the healthy shoulder

9. They work and do the same thing

10. Now you have a peripheral image of both shoulders

This is your internal image of the affected shoulder, of how the white joint looks and the muscles and the tendons of what is in the picture. But, as you picture these places on the shoulder, also picture the affected shoulder being a healthy working shoulder, because you have this attached picture of a healthy shoulder. Now, you have a healthy shoulder on the affected side, that can work, and you have a colorful image to follow as a guide for how it works.

You have your internal image of the affected shoulder now, the one that is on the picture. It is one that has a white shoulder joint, with smooth muscles on the joint, and red tendons, that look healthy. You have this picture in your head of how the inside of the affected shoulder looks, and now you can think of it when you want, as often as you want, and know that you have an internal image of the affected shoulder that you can compare to the healthy shoulder.

As you think of this internal image more often, you will begin to form a memory of thinking that the affected shoulder has a round joint, smooth muscles and tendons, and assume that it works.

This association becomes your new internal image and one that you will use each time you think of the affected shoulder. You will be able to use this internal image when you are picturing the affected shoulder working, such as when you need to reach for items.

Example 4.5: Use the picture of the internal image to form a peripheral image of both shoulders (use for 2x day)

1. Stand at the kitchen counter

2. Wear your patch

3. Keep eyes lowered to the counter

4. Try to imagine how you looked in the shirt in the mirror

5. Picture how the chest looks in the shirt

6. Try keeping this image in your thoughts

7. Imagine how the healthy arm looks out of the side of your eyes.

8. Imagine how the affected arm looks out of the side of your eyes

9. Now, try to picture how the chest, shoulders, and arms look all at once out of the corners of your eyes

10. Glance down at the affected shoulder if you need to.

11. This is your peripheral image of the upper body

12. Take a rest.

This is an intentional exercise and one that allows you to show that you are including the two shoulders in the image – though one is a patch.

Planning to look at the shoulders and arms as a peripheral image is the same type of action that you would do if you were standing at the kitchen counter yourself and were planning to reach for a glass. The idea that you decided to keep the picture of how you looked in the shirt in the mirror, in your thoughts, and then include both images of the upper arms and shoulders in the peripheral image, is a purposeful gesture, and one that the mirror cells will take notice of, even if the image is missing some of the internal image of the shoulder and the hand.

Exercise 4.6: Attach a memory of how the picture looks to the affected shoulder (Use for 1x day)

1. Stand in one place
2. Study how the shoulder, smooth muscles and the tendons look in the picture
3. Do this for a minute
4. As you do this, you are associating the picture with the shoulders
5. Then look down at the shoulders
6. Imagine that the shoulder joint, smooth muscles and tendons look the same
7. Then look straight ahead
8. Imagine that both shoulders have this same white smooth shoulder joint, smooth muscles and red tendons.
9. As you do this, you may picture how both shoulders look with this white shoulder joint, and smooth muscles and tendons

The picture is a substitute for this feeling, but one that does work, because it shows the parts of the shoulder that you would normally think about, only in a different way.

Checkpoint: Do peripheral exercises for 3-4 weeks, 2x day. Work on being able to include the affected arm in the peripheral image of the two sides. Glimpse down at the picture on the affected shoulder and walk around with it on as often as you can, to try to imagine that you need both shoulders and that the affected one works as well as the healthy one.

Chapter 5: Reach with a short rehearsal

This move is needed if you have tried to form the thought of having a plan but can't keep the thought for more than few seconds or recall how the affected shoulder looks in the image.

As you recall, mirror cells need to absorb this peripheral image, but to do this, they need for the image to look the same on both sides.

In this case, you need to find a way to demonstrate the move to attract mirror cells, rather than try to get the peripheral image to look the right way.

With practice the image will improve, but for now, you are more interested in what this memory that returns from the mirror cells is doing, and how you can use it to think through the motion.

Showing what you plan to do, in the form of four short handshakes, attracts mirror cells, and brings back the memory of how you used to reach with your hand. If you use a memory of how to reach with your hand, then you will be using your hand exactly as you usually do, and this will reinforce the absorption process for the activity in the brain.

Steps for rehearsal:

1. Point the eyes down toward the counter and keep them in this position.

2. Point handshake hand toward the item that you want to reach

3. Bring handshake hand and arm forward five inches.

4. Shake the healthy hand four times in a row toward the cup.

   This is four seconds, one second per shake.

5. The reach memory returns, and now you are more aware of the shoulders.

The handshake position:

- Turn healthy hand on its side
- Keep fingers straight, but loose
- Thumb is straight

This activity is four seconds, divided into four shakes. So, this will be one shake, two shakes, three shakes, four shakes, and then you are done. It is only four seconds of shakes, and then the memory of how to hold the hand and the shoulders returns.

Steps for reach:

1. The memory returns of how to hold the shoulders.
2. Swing the affected hand up, in front of you, four inches from the chin.
3. Hold arm in place.
4. Keep eyes pointed down toward the counter
5. Focus on how the affected shoulder feels
6. Say drop and relax if need to
7. Begin to reach out your hand.

Your thoughts should be on the peripheral image that is in place, that you created when you performed the handshake rehearsal. Then you want to turn your attention to the internal image you have of the affected shoulder.

Exercise 5.0: Shake the hand to attract a memory of how to reach out the hand (use for 2x day)

1. Stand at counter
2. Hold arms in the swing position

3. Keep eyes pointed down at the counter in front of the cup

4. Point handshake hand toward the cup

5. Bring arm and handshake hand forward five inches

6. Shake handshake hand four times toward the cup

7. The memory of how to use the shoulder and hand returns

8. Lift affected hand up

9. Pause

10. Say "drop and relax," to lower joint into the socket

11. Stay focused on the affected shoulder

12. Then slowly reach out the hand toward the item.

Mirror cells accept this handshake position as a possible way to reach for an item, because you are holding the hand in the same position as you would if you were going to reach for an item – hand on the side, with fingers held loosely.

The position of the eyes is the same too, as when you form the peripheral image, preparing to reach for items – pointed down – so you can see both arms and hands, in the image, while you are preparing to reach, and then as you reach out the hand.

Joint into the socket:

1. Pause

2. Say "drop and relax."

3. Picture the joint falling into the socket

4. Extend your hand.

Drop and relax allows you to adjust the shoulder the same way you usually would, and make the action look like how you would normally adjust the shoulder. This makes the action the same as how you would adjust the healthy shoulder, and so this is another way to bring the two peripheral images of the upper body together in one image.

The swing position: This is when you hold your arms in a loose bent position at your sides and can swing them back and forth is you need to.

Exercise 5.1: Acquiring the peripheral image and internal image of the shoulders during rehearsal (use for 2x day)

1. Stand at the counter
2. Hold arms in the swing position
3. Keep eyes pointed down at the counter in front of cup
4. Point handshake hand toward the cup
5. Bring pointed hand forward five inches
6. Shake handshake hand four times toward the cup
7. As you finish the fourth shake, you will notice that you have more focus on the shoulders. (peripheral image)
8. Switch over to the affected side
9. Swing affected hand up (internal image)

As soon as you finish with the rehearsal then you have a memory of needing to hold the shoulders in place. You also get back an internal image for the affected shoulder. This allows you to form an image of how the shoulder joint works and the muscles if you can identify with how the inside of the shoulder looks.

Use rehearsal to lift the hand up to the mouth:

This works the same way as normal reach, except that you need to use the handshake hand four times in a row, up to your mouth, rather than a normal reach.

Example: Reach the hand up to mouth

1. Stand at the counter
2. Hold arms in the swing position
3. Keep eyes angled down slightly so you can see the arm
4. Bring the healthy hand up to mouth four times in a row
5. Then start to lift the affected hand up to the mouth
6. Pause
7. Say drop and relax
8. Finish bringing the hand up to the mouth

This may take a few tries, to get the shoulder to adjust this way, because the joint is adjusting as you bring the elbow inward toward the stomach, but the peripheral image is strong for this activity and so you will be able to keep an eye on how you are looking at the arm and shoulder.

Exercise 5.2 Practice reaching the hand up to the mouth (use for 2x a day)

1. Stand at the counter
2. Hold arms in the swing position
3. Keep eyes angled down slightly so you can see the arm
4. Bring the healthy hand up to the mouth four times in a row
5. Then start to lift the affected hand up to the mouth

6. Pause

7. Say drop and relax

8. Finish bringing the hand up to the mouth

The eyes should be angled down the same way as they were when you reached for the cup. This is because whenever you reach up to the mouth, or across for an item, you need to keep the arms and hands in your peripheral vision.

Checkpoint: do the exercises 2x a day for three weeks. The rehearsal exercises can be done any amount of times that you need because you are always providing the reach image to the brain.

Chapter 6: Rehearse for a hand memory

If you were to rehearse how to open a door, the task would be the same – reach out the hand four times in a row, open the door – and the memory of how to open the door would then be returned. The movements stay the same no matter where you reach, or what you are reaching for, and to this is the part that the mirror cells have a memory for, rather than the specific part of when you grab the doorknob.

Mirror cells don't have a specific memory of how the hand turns a doorknob, because this is considered grabbing, rather than turning, and the grabbing motion is the same as one that you would use to grab a glass, or plate, of a door handle. Notice that after you grab the door handle, you are simply holding onto the doorknob, and then turning, it with some wrist motion.

This is because the doorknob itself, is not something you retrieve, but hold onto so you can open the door. The fingers are only made to grab things, and hold them in place, and so there wouldn't be any other motion attached to how you open a door.

The mirror cells do know how to reach, however, and they do this well, and there is only one position that you can hold the hand and arm for reach. So, when you reach for a doorknob, or anything else, the motions are the same, placing the arm in a bent position, and then pointing the hand toward the item that you need, and then grab onto the doorknob.

The car:

Placing your hand on a steering wheel gives you back the same kind of reach memory you would get if you were to reach for a door knob or a cup on a counter. The only difference is that you are reaching up to your hands in a shorter-range motion. This motion is only a few inches away from the target, which is the wheel, but you have the same plan, to rehearse on one side, and then follow through with the motion on the other side.

Steps to rehearsing placing hands on the steering wheel:

1. Keep eyes looking straight ahead, at the top of the wheel, across to dash
2. Make sure you can see both hands out of corners of eyes.
3. Lift healthy hand up along one side of the wheel four times in a row. (memory).
4. Keep the healthy hand on the wheel.
5. Bring the affected hand up along the other side of the steering wheel and leave the hand in this position for several seconds.
6. Feel the position of the hand on the wheel, and the tension at the front of the upper arm.
7. Feel the muscles working on the arm and shoulder.

The reach motion on the healthy side was for four seconds. Then the reach up of the affected hand was only once because the memory was working.

Exercise 6.0: Practice bringing your hand up along the wheel four times in a row. (use this 1x day)

1. Lift healthy hand up on wheel four times in a row (memory returns)
2. Bring affected hand up on wheel once, and leave it in this position
3. Notice the angle that you hold the shoulder
4. And the tension at the front of the shoulder
5. Notice that you are more attentive to the affected hand now and can feel the muscles working in the chest region, which is next to the shoulder.

This rehearsal can be done a few times in a row

A door handle:

Opening a cabinet door, or any door with a handle, such as a refrigerator door, a door leading into a building, or a sliding door, requires the same action, and one that you can use the reach rehearsal.

In this case, you are using the hand the same way but in a slightly different angle. You might be pointing your hand up toward a cabinet door, or grabbing the handle differently, such as with a sliding cup door. Though the angles are different, the motions are the same, and there is no variation in how you do the rehearsal motion.

Steps to grabbing a door handle:

1. Stand in front of the door handle (refrigerator, cabinet)
2. Keep eyes lowered toward refrigerator door
3. Bring healthy arm forward five inches
4. Bring the hand up four times in a row toward the handle
5. Bring affected hand up to grab the door handle.
6. Open the door

In this case, you reached up to shake the healthy hand at the door handle. And then you reached up again to grab the door handle with your other hand. Notice that you brought the healthy arm forward five inches, as you would if you were reaching for a cup on a counter.

Drop and relax can still be used for any type of reach rehearsal, and the steps are the same. You will say, "Drop and relax," command, as you start to reach out the shoulder on the affected side.

So, then the steps are:

1. Stand in front of the door handle

2. Bring healthy arm forward five inches

3. Bring your hand up four times in a row toward the handle

4. Start to reach your affected hand up toward the handle

5. Pause

6. Focus on the location of the joint in the affected shoulder

7. Say, "Drop and relax."

8. Bring the other hand up to grab the door handle.

9. Open the door

The pause arrives after you begin to lift the affected hand up, in front of you, and then you take a few seconds or a minute to study how the shoulder feels.

Exercise 6.0: Reach for the refrigerator door handle:

1. Stand in front of the refrigerator door

2. Lower eyes to the refrigerator door

3. Point healthy hand-shake hand in direction of the door

4. Shake hand four times in a row

5. Switch to affected hand

6. Lift the hand

7. Pause

8. Think of the internal image of the shoulder

9. Say "drop, and relax," as you are still thinking of the shoulder

10. Then reach out the hand toward the door of the refrigerator

Exercise 6.1: Reach for a dish out of the drain:

1. Stand in front of the refrigerator door

2. Point eyes down to dish drain

3. Point healthy hand-shake hand toward dish drain

4. Shake hand four times in a row

5. Switch to affected hand

6. Lift the hand

7. Pause

8. Think of the internal image of the shoulder

9. Say "drop, and relax," as you are still thinking of the shoulder

10. Bring hand forward slowly

11. Then reach out the hand toward the dish in the drain

Drop and relax works when you are out too, such as in a grocery store, or in a restaurant. This is done on a much smaller scale because you are in a crowded environment, but you can still get it done, by reaching out the hand more subtly, and then saying "drop and relax, "to yourself, rather than out loud.

Exercise 6.2: Drop and relax in the grocery store (use as needed)

1. Stand in front of the shelf

2. Look straight ahead at the item that you need on the shelf

3. Shake your hand four times toward the item.

4. Try to think of the shoulders

5. One shoulder will feel and look different than the other one

6. Try and picture the bare shoulder on the affected side

7. Say "drop and relax."

8. Imagine that the shoulder joint drops down into the socket.

9. You should know this feeling when it does

10. After a few seconds, reach out your hand to the item.

Checkpoint: There is no time limit for these exercises because they will be needed often. As you recover and get back that feeling of knowing how the shoulder is made, and what it is doing, and how well you can picture it in your head, you will have to return to these exercises at least once a day, to check the position of the shoulder, and see how you are supposed to be using the shoulder and hand.

Chapter 7: Reach with a peripheral image

This is when you start to transition from using reach and rehearsal to trying to use a peripheral image on your own. You will work off a memory of how the shirt looks in the mirror and noticing the pattern of the shirt and how the shoulders look in the shirt, so you can recreate this at the sink. Then you need to be able to hold onto a memory of how the shoulders and arms looked in the mirror and try to picture this in your head as you plan to reach for the item on the counter.

Steps:

1. Stand at counter

2. Try to picture yourself in the patterned shirt

3. Visualize seeing the chest area of the patterned shirt

4. And how the shoulders look

5. Try to hold onto this image in your head

6. Look down at the hands

7. Imagine that you need both hands the same way

8. Look over at the glass

9. Angle eyes down toward counter

10. Then keep thinking of the position of the shoulders and arms.

11. Lift affected hand slowly

12. Pause.

13. Think of having to adjust the shoulder joint (drop and relax if needed)

14. After a few seconds start to reach out the hand toward the glass.

You'll want to focus on the details of the shirt, such as the thick trim border on the shirt, and a detailed pattern on the chest portion of the shirt. This will improve your chances of retaining the chest image, and upper arms as you try to form the peripheral image.

Exercise 7.0: Face the mirror to study how the patterned shirt looks (use this 2x day)

1. Face the mirror in the patterned shirt
2. Study how you look in the shirt.
3. Notice the shape of the neckline
4. The detailed pattern of the shirt
5. The thick green border of the shirt
6. Notice the details on the shirt-sleeves
7. Notice how the shoulders and chest look at one time
8. Leave the mirror and rest.

The internal image of the affected shoulder is still off slightly, and you are only able to form what you know so far, which is how the shoulder joint looks, and how the tension feels at the front of the shoulder. This is enough for you to form some of the peripheral image of the affected side, but a better way is to be able to feel the tension at the front of the shoulders and look at how the round part of the shoulders looks in the short-sleeve shirt at the same time in the mirror.

Exercise 7.1: Try and feel the internal image of the shoulders (use this 2x day)

1. Leave the mirror
2. Stand at the counter
3. Lower your eyes so you can see both arms and hands

4. Focus on how the two shoulders feel

5. Focus on the tension at the front of the shoulders

6. Try to feel the nudge of the shoulders joint against the skin

7. Swing the arms in place if you need to, to make sure aligned.

8. Try to keep this image of how the shoulders feel away from the mirror in your thoughts

9. Try to think of how the shoulders look. Are both aligned?

10. Do you feel the same tension on both shoulders?

11. If you do, then you have an internal image of the shoulders

12. If you don't then you may need rehearsal to study the feeling in the shoulders. Remember, the internal image is either a feeling of how the shoulders look or a picture of how they look and work.

An internal image of the shoulders that you should picture is one of associating a feeling that the muscles around the shoulder joint are in place, and that this means that the shoulder joint is in the right place. So, from the nudging feeling at the front of the shoulder, you should be building up to a feeling of a large muscle over the shoulder joint, that you picture working, and being able to use on both shoulders.

Now, you can use the swing position, to try to secure that tension feeling in both shoulders, but when you do, imagine that there is the round joint, and the feeling of the thick shoulder muscle in place at the same time.

Exercise 7.2: Face the mirror to test out the swing position of the shoulders (use this 2x day)

1. Face the mirror in the patterned shirt

2. Study the outline of the round part of the shoulders in the shirt.

3. Swing the arms in place, and see how the round part of the shoulder feels

4. On the sixth swing, halt

5. Study how the shoulders feel in this position.

6. Study how the shoulders look in the shirt-sleeve in the mirror.

Next, you need to try to picture in your head how the shoulders look from a front view. Think back to when you were in front of the mirror a few minutes ago. How did you look in the shirt? How do you think the shoulder looked beneath the shirt sleeve?

If you can't draw on this memory, then return to the mirror and try to examine the shoulders again in the patterned short-sleeve shirt. Stay in front of the mirror for up to a minute, examining the outline of how the shoulders look on the affected shirt-sleeve.

Exercise 7.3: Practice looking down at the peripheral image of the upper body (use this for 2x day)

1. Stand in front of the mirror in the patterned shirt.

2. Look at how the shoulders look in the patterned shirt

3. Swing arms in place

4. Try to feel the tension in the shoulder joints

5. Halt after the sixth swing

6. Hold the arms in the swing position.

7. Walk over the kitchen counter.

8. Lower your eyes to the counter.

9. Picture how the shoulders and arms look out of the corners of your eyes.

10. Swing them slightly so you can see them better in the image.

11. Try to picture how the front of the shirt looks.

12. Try to hang onto these images for a few seconds.

The image should be of the two shoulders in the patterned shirt, and the arms and hands, as you would see it from a front view as if you were looking at yourself. You should picture the front view in the shirt that you have on already, or are wearing today, so peripheral images change based on what you are wearing, but the position of the shoulders and chest never changes, or the feeling that you are supposed to have in the shoulders and the upper arms in the same position each time you form the peripheral image.

Exercise 7.4: Study how the shoulders look from a front view at the counter (Use this 2x day)

1. Study the outline of the shoulders in the shirt in the mirror

2. Try to feel the tension in front of the shoulders

3. Try to feel that nudge of the shoulder up against the skin

4. Swing the arms to feel the tension

5. Leave the mirror, head to the counter

6. Hold arms in the swing position

7. Keep eyes down toward the counter

8. You should see the shoulders, arms and, hands out of the corners of your eyes.

9. Try to picture how the shirt looks from a front view, such as a boat-necked collar, or a thick seamed edging.

10. Try to keep this image of how the shirt looks from a front view in your thoughts for a few seconds

The image of the shirt should be a memory, but if you are still having trouble remembering how you looked in it, return to the mirror to study the front view of the chest, shoulders and upper arms before going to the counter.

Exercise 7.5: Identity of shoulders and arms, imagine that you need to reach (use for 2x day)

1. Stand in front of the mirror for up to a minute.
2. Take in the image of the shirt and shoulders
3. Swing arms, to remind yourself of the location of the tension at the front of the shoulder.
4. Walk to the counter
5. Lower eyes
6. Picture the shoulders, arms and hands in the image (peripheral)
7. Try to picture how the front of the shirt looks (boat neck, scooped)
8. Try to hang onto these two images in your thoughts for two minutes
9. Keep thinking of how the front of the shirt looks
10. Keep holding arms in swing position.
11. Imagine that you need to use your affected hand to reach for the cup.

The reach of the hand is closely associated with how the muscles in the shoulder look and work. This can be shown, by the need for the front image of how you look at your shirt, and chest, in the peripheral image, for up to one minute.

So, when you approach the counter and lower your eyes, you are picturing the peripheral image of the two arms and hands, off to the side of the eyes, and the feeling of the shoulders being in place, but this is not enough for the mirror cells to allow you to reach out the hand. You still need the hand and internal image of the affected shoulder.

The mirror as a reminder:

The mirror returns a reflective memory to you of how you are supposed to be thinking through the tasks. This is done quickly, so you can stand in front of the mirror, remind yourself of the motion, and then be back at the sink or counter in just a few minutes.

In front of the mirror, pretend that you are reaching out your hand as you normally would at the counter, and focus on how the affected shoulder feels. You will notice that you keep the shoulder in place more and that the tension is noticeable on the affected shoulder. Notice any adjustments you make to the shoulders to keep them in place, such as relaxing the shoulder muscles or bringing the joint forward a few inches, and the elbow in toward the stomach a half an inch. This is to get you to hold the arm and shoulder in the right place.

The mirror delivers a memory to you of how to inspect the shoulder and arm, but also how to make changes to how you are holding the arm, instantly, because you are now focusing on the peripheral image you see in the mirror, and the memory tells you what to adjust based on how the shoulders feel.

The memory gives you back internal images of the shoulders, and how they are supposed to feel and look. So, you are simply following along with what the memory is telling you to do.

Any of these feelings in the muscles are more noticeable on the affected side because the brain is learning how to accept this image again for the first time. You're using motor functions to move these muscles, and so it will feel like you're using them for the first time.

After a few reaches, of analyzing how you are holding the shoulders while you reach, and studying the position of the shoulders, return to the counter and try to keep the shoulders in this position. Try to focus on the tension at the front of the shoulder, and how you are holding the arm. Then try to reach for the glass.

How to create a peripheral image in front of the mirror:

1. Stand in front of the mirror
2. Study how shoulders look
3. After about four to ten seconds, you suddenly know how to hold the shoulders.
4. It's obvious that you need to adjust the shoulder or arm
5. You feel as if you in control of your movements.

You can do this as often as you need to, and for as long as you need to, because the mirror attracts mirror cells right away, and you get the memory back that you need to use for the activity.

Checkpoint: Keep doing the exercises for three weeks, 2x day. You may need to work on, some of the aspects of being able to form the entire peripheral image, such as the identity of the shoulders, and imagining that both shoulders and arms look and work the same way in the patterned shirt. You may also need to work on holding the image in your thoughts of how the shoulders and chest look, for longer than three minutes. The next chapter on the hand will give you that missing piece of the peripheral image you need, which is to bring back the memory of how to look at the hand.

Chapter 8: The hands and forearms

The hand image is different than of the other motor parts, because they aren't used to supporting any weight, or present a certain appearance for the peripheral image to attract mirror cells.

These creates a need to be able to recognize them another way, other than studying of the bones and muscles look and feel.

The characteristics of how they look, as well as planned motions based on memories attracts mirror cells, and has you closely examining how they work nearly every few seconds of the day.

This is when you begin to analyze how you hold the hands and how the shape of the knuckles tells you when you are holding the fingers in a delicate curve and if this position matches how you held them in the past and if you like how you are holding them.

So, the pattern is, to study how the hands look, so that you can attract mirror cells, provided you recognize the characteristics of the hands. Then mirror cells absorb the image and bring back motor functions, and skills that you need to evaluate the shape of the knuckles. This allows you to examine how you hold the fingers and find a position that you want to hold them that suits you, based on a memory that returns from the mirror cells absorbing the image.

The characteristics:

These are any feature of the hands that you are used to seeing that tell you that these hands are yours. This includes the tone of the skin, such as the pale pink tone, or beige tone with a ruddy appearance. This is also defined by the lines you see on the hands, such as the crevices that you see between, the base, of the index finger and thumb. Or the shape of the thumb.

Traits also include how you are holding the hand, which can be lightly, heavily, or firmer, depending on your personality, and how well you can inflect decision making into how you hold the hand.

This all starts with needing to study how the hand and fingers look and use that intent approach to define the tasks, so the brain feels that you have a task planned with the hands.

Steps to comparing the hands:

1. Sit in a chair
2. Turn the healthy hand with palm up
3. Study the palm.
4. Notice the lines
5. The skin, tone
6. Notice that you expect the hand to work
7. Do this for a minute
8. Switch to the affected hand
9. Turn palm over with same expectations
10. Look at the lines
11. The skin, tone
12. Believe that you expect the hand to work
13. Now look down at both palms
14. Do this for one minute

The admiration for the hand is what the mirror cells want to see, to bring you back to the line of thinking you had before you were injured. Before the injury, admiring the hands, and knowing and thinking about all the traits was a typical procedure.

These expectations of how the hands and forearms should work, are the way you used to think when you looked at the hands and knew that they would work well during tasks.

The mirror cells want to see more of this kind of thinking, and this all starts with wanting to look at the traits of the hands, and identifying with them, to bring back this memory of how you used to decide how to use them, and recognize that how you move them, is the same way you moved them in the past.

Exercise 8.0 Restore a memory, of when you looked down at the knuckles of the hand. (Use for 2x a day)

1. Look down at the top of the healthy hand
2. Notice the lines on the wrist and knuckles at the base of fingers
3. Notice the lines at the top of the hands
4. Notice that these lines at the knuckles define how you hold the hand
5. You are more careful with how you hold the hand
6. Notice that you choose to hold the fingers a certain way
7. Straighten the hand, and then start to relax it, to study how the knuckles look.
8. Now, do the same on the affected hand
9. Imagine that these knuckles are also what defines this hand
10. Straighten and relax the fingers, to see the slight image of the knuckles
11. Notice the wrinkles around the knuckles

12. Turn the fingers down and notice the shape of them.

13. Take a rest

These knuckles and how they change shape, as you move them, are a memory that you have of how you looked at them in the past. This is the most significant memory of how you look at the hand from the top view, which defines how the hands look and is the most closely related memory to how you care about the hand and wanting to move the fingers a certain way.

Needing to look at the hands a certain way, and feeling like you need to use them, is a purposeful gesture, that shows the brain that you need the hand as much as you do the healthy one and returns you to the line of thinking that you had before the injury.

Exercise 8.1: Work on studying the tops of the hands (use for 2x day)

1. Start on the healthy side.

2. Look down at how the tops of the hands look

3. Look down at how the tops of the forearms look

4. Run your fingers across the forearm of the healthy hand

5. Say, "This forearm works well."

6. Then admire how the top of the healthy hand looks

7. Notice the skin tone, and lines and wrinkles

8. Switch to the affected hand

9. Notice the tops of the hands

10. And the skin tone

11. Run your fingers across the top of the forearm

12. Say, "I need this arm as much as the other one."

13. Admire the skin tone, and the lines and wrinkles

14. Say, "I need this hand as much as the other one."

Traits that you admire on this hand include wrinkles, the tone of skin, and the shape of the hand, and fingers, and a memory of how you want to hold the hand based on how the fingers are shaped.

The mirror cells absorbed the traits you saw on the healthy hand, and so when you get to the affected hand, many of the memories that you need to use for the task are already in place, you simply have to be able to show this need portion of the task, and the fact that you have a plan.

The forearm is used in this example because this is the part of the arm that you notice when you are looking at the hands and is always in your peripheral image. So, when you are trying to tell the brain that you are memorizing how the hand looks and the skin ton, you want to include this image in your thoughts as well.

Exercise 8.2: Study the hand from side to side

1. Stand for this exercise

2. Keep arms bent.

3. Look down at the healthy hand

4. Turn it so the palm is facing down

5. Notice that the wrist is steady

6. Say, "This hand works well."

7. Turn hand so palm is up.

8. Study lines

9. Say, "this hand is strong and able to move,"

10. Do this for a minute

11. Then switch to the affected side

12. Hold hand so palm faces down

13. Say, "This hand also works well."

14. Study how the skin looks

15. Believe that you are looking at a working hand

16. Turn hand over so palm is up

17. Say, "This hand also works well."

As you say these things, take note of how you admire how the top of the hand looks and feels, and the lines, and how you feel the hand and arm work as well, notice how steady this hand is, and how well you keep the wrist in place.

Also, the hands are very closely associated with measuring the timing of the tasks, and space, examining textures, and how things feel, to make decisions and assign meaning to the item that you are examining.

The fingertips for example, can be used for measuring how things look, so you can make decisions about the quality of an item, and what you think of the item.

Measuring if you want to use something is usually based on texture, but it is also based on your opinion of the surface area, such as a countertop, or a coffee table. An example of weaving opinion into examining a surface is running your fingers along the smooth surface of a laptop, and determining the quality of the laptop, and what you think of the style.

If you have your thumb along the edge of the screen, and the tips of the fingers along the top of the laptop, where the silver textured side, you will be examining how you feel about the surface of the top of the laptop.

Suppose this laptop has a ridged silver texture, so you can run fingertips starting at one corner and up one edge, then across the top, and then down the other side, to get a scope of how the surface of the whole top of the laptop feels.

The results are that the first side, where you brought your fingertips up to the corner, was ridged, as was the other side, but the top was smooth. This made you think that the top was slightly worn and that the edges sturdy. This may have made you think that the laptop was a slightly older model, based on the ridged surface. This is your opinion based on when you ran your fingertips along the edges of the laptop: that it is a slightly older model laptop.

Exercise 8.3: Study the characteristics of the hand (use this 2x day)

1. Stand or sit

2. Begin to look at the top of the healthy hand

3. Study the lines in the skin

4. How the thumb is shaped

5. The wrinkles on the knuckles

6. Notice how straight you keep the wrist

7. Do this for a minute

8. Now, switch, and look at the affected hand

9. Start, by noticing how the top of the hand looks

10. Say, "I need this hand just as much."

11. Notice the skin tone of the top of the hand

12. Notice the wrinkles on the knuckles

13. Take a rest

Exercise 8.4: Admire how the healthy hand looks and then the affected hand (use for 2x day)

1. Hold the healthy hand out in front of you as if you are admiring a ring

2. Notice the shape of the hand

3. Notice how you are holding the fingers

4. Look at how the wrist bends up

5. Admire how the forearm looks

6. Run your fingers along the skin of the forearm

7. Notice the crevices between the thumb and the bottom of the index finger

8. Hold out your affected hand the same way

9. Try admiring the hand the same way

10. Try holding the fingers the same way

11. Imagine that you need to look at this hand the same way

12. Touch the skin of the hand and forearm

13. Say "this skin looks the same as the other hand and arm,"

This next exercise teaches you how to plan out moves in advance of moving the hand. First, you'll think through how to plan to move the hand. Then work through in your mind, the steps to bringing the affected fingers over to the other hand to retrieve the bottle.

Exercise 8.5: Exchange a bottle between hands (use for 2x day)

1. Sit in a chair

2. Hold a pint-size bottle in the healthy hand

3. Do this for a few seconds

4. Form a plan for the affected hand to receive the bottle

5. Bring the bottle over to the affected hand

6. Then bring it back over to the healthy hand

7. Watch how you grab the bottle as you bring it over to the healthy hand

8. How did you prepare the hand to receive the bottle?

9. Place the bottle in the healthy hand

10. When did the hand move?

11. Did you anticipate accepting the bottle ahead of time?

12. Did you bring the hand over to the affected hand?

13. Try to create the same motions with the affected side hand when you accept the bottle.

This is an exercise in anticipation of the visual images you need to create of the healthy hand before you place the bottle in the palm of this hand. First, you need to picture needing to use the hand, so mirror cells react. Then you need to picture the task and to decide if you will bring the healthy hand over to the affected hand, to retrieve the bottle, or wait to place the bottle in the palm of the affected hand. Then you need to imagine how the healthy hand will look when you reach for the bottle.

These images start with looking at the healthy hand for a minute, before you get started, and picturing the task that you need to do in your head. This allows you to identify with how the hand looks for a minute, and since it is the healthy hand that you are identifying with first, the mirror cells will absorb this image quickly. Which is why you start on the healthy hand.

The planning portion of the task, of now needing to pass the bottle over to the affected hand, takes the most effort because now you need the affected hand as much as you do the healthy one. Take a minute to imagine this.

Exercise 8.6 Practice needing the affected hand as much as the healthy one (use for 2x)

1. Hold the water bottle in the healthy hand
2. Do this for a minute
3. You will be able to see the affected hand
4. Imagine that you need this affected hand as much as you do the healthy hand
5. Look down at the slightly cupped affected hand for a minute
6. You are anticipating having to use it
7. Imagine that you can take this bottle out of the healthy hand and try to picture these moves in your head.
8. Practice bringing the fingers over to the healthy hand
9. Bring the fingertips together and pull them back as if you are grabbing a piece of yarn.
10. Pull in a tugging motion.
11. This allows you to recreate the motion of bringing something toward you

So, now you have worked out some of the motions you need to reach the fingers over and grab the water bottle, which is a task and gives the hand a purpose. The mirror cells will notice that you have reached the fingers over to the healthy side and done so in a similar way you may have in the past, and so this action brings the two hands more closely together in the image. This is also showing intent in the action that you plan to use the affected hand to reach over and get the bottle.

Exercise 8.7: Practice showing that you have a purpose with the affected hand (use for 2x a day)

1. Hold the bottle in the healthy hand.

2. Bring fingers on the affected side, over to opposite hand

3. Use the spider formation of the fingers, as if you are pulling a piece of yarn

4. Tug on this yarn a second

5. Then bring the hand back

6. Return to cupped formation

   Tug on this yarn several times in a row. Do the exercise a few more times

   The need aspect is apparent when you rehearse to bring the hand over to the bottle. Now, you have shown that you need this hand, and can walk through the activity that you plan. So, now it seems more realistic that you would be able to reach your hand over to get the bottle out of the healthy hand.

Exercise 8.8: Reach for the bottle with your affected hand (use for 2x a day)

1. Hold the bottle in the healthy hand

2. Pull the yarn, four times, with your affected hand

3. Then reach for the bottle out of the healthy hand

4. Hold it for a minute in the palm of the affected hand.

   The weight of the bottle will create an image of how the palm feels when there is something against the skin. These sensations, of feeling weight, and the cold of the bottle, as well as the label, allow you to measure the importance of the item in the palm of the hand, create an image of it, and then determine how long you want to keep it in the palm of your hand. These are all decisions that you would normally make about the bottle after you acquire it, such as deciding how long you will hold the bottle, if you should drink the water, if you want to turn your hand on the side and hold the bottle this way, or if you want to put the water bottle down. Any of these will finish the task, and then you can move onto another one.

Bringing back a memory of how you looked at the hand and the fingers, can be done by studying how the hand looks and feels. Add in a texture element, such as a soft tissue, and now you have the brain working to try to bring back the memories you need to get back of needing to define the hands, and memories that return of the past, and how you looked in the past.

How to hold the hand for the tissue exercise:

1. Form a loose fist with fingers gently curled
2. Turn fist on side and keep fingers gently curled, and hovering over the palm of the hand
3. Make sure you can still see the fingernails.
4. Rest thumb on the first knuckle of the index finger
5. Place a folded square piece of soft tissue under the thumb, and rest thumb gently against the knuckle of the index finger.

Exercise 8.9: Study how the thumbnail and skin look with the square tissue (use for 2x day)

This is a two-minute exercise and is designed for you to examine the hand slowly.

1. Turn loose fist on the side, so the thumb is facing you
2. Make sure thick, square piece of tissue is under the thumb
3. Study how the thumbnail is shaped
4. Notice the shape of the thumb
5. Keep looking at the thumbnail for ten seconds
6. Turn the loose fist gently, so you look at the fingernails

7. Look at how the thumb muscle is shaped

8. Notice the lines on the palm

9. Do this for ten seconds.

10. Then turn hand so looking at the top of the hand

11. Keep fingers curled

12. Notice the lines on the top of the hand

13. Notice the skin tone

14. Notice how the knuckles are shaped.

15. Take a rest

This is the cognitive section of the brain start to work, as well as the perception and recognition portions of the brain because you have been looking at the hand in a way, that shows purpose and the same way you normally would for tasks.

You may also have felt some recognition in the arm and shoulder, as well, because looking at the hand brings back a memory of holding the shoulder and arm in place as well.

Exercise 8.10: Study how the thumbnail and skin look with the square tissue (use for 2x day)

Examine the hand slowly.

1. Turn loose fist on the side, so the thumb is facing you

2. Make sure thick, square piece of tissue is under the thumb

3. Study how the thumbnail is shaped

4. Notice the shape of the thumb

5. Do this for ten seconds.

6. Then turn hand so you can see the palm of the hand

7. Study how the fingernails look

8. Notice the shape of them

9. How each one is different

10. Do this for ten seconds

11. Then turn hand back to thumb

12. Keep studying the thumb for ten seconds.

13. Then turn hand so you are looking at the top of the hand

14. Do this for ten seconds.

15. Take a rest

This takes a few days of doing this tissue exercise, to be able to start to notice that you have improved concentration and feel more productive after you finish the exercise. This is a sign that you are absorbing some of the image of the hand, and that the mirror cells are noticing your diligence and persistence with the exercise mostly, of needing to look at the hand.

You may notice some memories of the past, returning too, such as how you used to study the fingernails, but not all the nails. This is a trace memory returning, of only a small amount of a memory returning, but not the whole thing.

A trace memory of the whole memory is not the entire memory or even a memory that is relevant to how you move the hand, or how you are supposed to be viewing the characteristics. It is usually a memory of when you looked at your nails years ago, and were sitting in a car, or park, or were a child and were looking down at the nail the exact same way you did in this exercise.

This memory is significant because it shows the memory of the hands returning, and this memory won't be of anything recent unless you have been practicing a lot in front of the mirror and looking down at your two sides in the peripheral vision.

Checkpoint: Do the hand exercises 2x a day, as needed. It is when you feel that you want to do the exercise, but at least once a day works, because this is enough time to generate brain activity for two hours. This is because hand exercises require a lot of planning, studying, and recognition, and so the brain needs to sort out these tasks that you tried to do. If you are recovering from a stroke, this will take at least two hours, because the brain processes image much slower when you are working with this kind of absorption of images.

Chapter 9: The legs and feet

The bottom of the feet, create sensations that tell you how to step, and these are used for other reasons as well. These sensations tell the mirror cells where you have your feet, and this allows you to visualize the placement of the feet and be aware of how the leg is moving.

This sensation can be used as a measure to define how you walk and tell the mirror cells about your activity. The more you feel these sensations at the bottom of the feet, the more you have control over how and where you place the feet.

These exercises work for someone that needs practice forming visual images when they walk and need to know how they are stepping. The sensations will give them the ability to study how they are walking in relation to the healthy side and use the motor functions and skills that return from the healthy side, to sort through the activity on their affected foot.

Exercise 9.0: Step to know how to place the feet (use for 2x a day)

1. Start with the healthy foot
2. Bring foot out to the side, and then step toe first
3. Start to count to four
4. Count 1,2,3,4
5. As you do, slowly bring the toe of the foot down, count 1,2, then the ball of the foot 3, and then the heel 4.
6. Place the foot firmly on the ground
7. Lean into foot a bit, to be able to detect how the bottom of the foot feels.
8. This creates awareness of the sensation at the bottom of the foot.

9. Then start on the affected foot.

10. Bring foot out to the side, then step toe first

11. Start to count to four.

12. Count 1,2,3,4

13. As you do, bring toe down slowly, count 1and 2 then lower the ball of the foot. Say 3, and then lower the heel to the floor. When place heel on floor, say 4.

14. Place the foot firmly on ground

15. Lean into foot a bit, to be able to detect how the bottom of the foot feels.

16. This creates awareness of the sensation at the bottom of foot.

Go back to the healthy foot and repeat steps. Do this until you have taken ten steps. Take a rest.

So the pressing down onto a flat surface with the healthy foot, will show you what you are supposed to be looking for, with the sensations at the bottom of the foot, and show you that pressing down onto the foot this way allows you to make decisions about the foot. Then you can repeat these steps on the affected foot slowly. The idea is that you will learn to recognize the sensations on the affected foot as well as you do the healthy foot.

These sensations are what allow you to create the peripheral image you need of the feet, without having to look down at them all the time. These sensations, or internal image of the feet, prompt you to create the visual image of the feet that you need to be able to recognize when you are walking the right way, and trigger the motor functions of the brain to return so you can use the motor skills you need to be able to perceive how the feet are placed on the floor.

This is also about needing to start to concentrate on how you are placing the foot on the ground, and the sensations at the bottom of the foot, and how the knee and leg look to you, as you are place them down on the surface of the floor, so you can plan how you will place the foot on the ground.

Exercise 9.1: Study effects of the sensations of the bottom of the healthy foot (use for 2x a day)

1. Start with the healthy foot
2. Bring foot out to the side, and then step toe first and then bend toes, and lean on them in this position.
3. Start to count to four
4. Count 1,2,3,4
5. As you do, bring toe down slowly, count 1 and 2. Then bring the ball of the foot down, count 3, and then land on heel, count 4. (like a dance routine)
6. Lean into foot a bit when placed flat on floor, with knee bent. Do this for five seconds.
7. This is to be able to detect how the bottom of the foot feels.
8. This creates awareness of the sensation at the bottom of foot.
9. Notice when you do lean, that you are also more aware of how the leg and ankle look and feel.
10. Notice as you lean, that you are more aware of the timing of the task, which is how long you want to take on the task.
11. Notice that the planning ability returns.
12. Notice that you start to picture your foot as you set it down
13. Take a rest

As you lean on the healthy foot you'll notice that you'll start to form plans of how long to stay on the foot, and how long you will do this on the other side. This is because you have created a peripheral image of seeing the foot, and lowering it to the floor, out of the corner of the eyes. This attracts mirror cells and allows them to return motor functions and skills that include planning, recognition and visual imaging of how the leg and foot look.

Exercise 9.2: Focus on the peripheral image of the feet (use for 2x a day)

1. Start with the healthy foot
2. Bring foot out to the side, and then step toe first
3. Notice that you can see the foot and leg out of the corners of your eyes.
4. This is the peripheral image of the feet.
5. Start to count to four
6. Count 1,2,3,4
7. As you do, bring toe down slowly, count 1and 2 then lower the ball of the foot. Say 3, and then lower the heel to the floor. When place heel on floor, say 4.
8. Place the foot firmly on the ground
9. Lean into foot a bit when placed flat on floor, with knee bent. Do this for five seconds.
10. This creates awareness of the sensation at the bottom of the foot.
11. Bring affected foot out to the side, and do the same
12. Step toe first
13. Try to see the foot out of the corners of your eyes
14. Try to imagine how the foot looks as you place the toes on the ground
15. Start to count to four.
16. Count 1,2,3,4
17. As you do, bring toe down slowly, count 1,2 , then the ball of the foot 3, and then the heel 4.
18. Place the foot firmly on ground
19. Lean into foot a bit, to be able to detect how bottom of foot feels.

20. This creates awareness of the sensation at the bottom of foot.

Step this way, ten times across the room.

Studying the toes for several seconds attracts mirror cells to your image because they think that you are going to walk. You have looked at your feet before you walked in the past, and so this image is in your memory, otherwise, it would not return after you have looked at the feet for several seconds.

Exercise 9.3: Study the toes for up to ten seconds (use for 2x day)

Wear sandals, or stand in bare feet so you can see the toes.

1. Find a threshold to stand in, on a flat surface
2. This is your starting point for potential walking
3. Make sure you can look straight ahead several yards, such as at a rug.
4. Stand with your feet a few inches apart
5. Make sure you can see the toes. (sandals)
6. Start on the healthy side and look down at the toes.
7. Start on the healthy foot, and count 1,2,3,4 as you look at the toes
8. Then jump over to the affected foot, count to 5,6,7,8 as you look at the toes
9. Then back at to the healthy side, and count to 9,10,11,12
10. Then back at the affected side and count to 13,14,15,16
11. Take a rest.

Make sure that the numbers are in consecutive order, and that there is no pausing between counting the numbers when you switch feet. So, the first foot, on the healthy side will be 1,2,3,4 then the foot on the affected side will be 5,6,7,8 and so on…because you can count to as high a number that you want.

Counting is a verbal prompt to attract mirror cells to you looking down at your feet. This keeps them focused on your feet image the whole time, and not other things you see, such as the hands.

Glancing up at the destination across the dining room, or over to where the green carpet is located, is a sign that you have a plan and tells the mirror cells that you have another plan in mind besides looking down at the feet and looking at the toes.

Exercise 9.4: Count while looking at toes, and look up at the destination (use for 2x day)

1. Stand in the threshold
2. Find a threshold to stand in, on a flat surface
3. This is your starting point for potential walking
4. Make sure you can look straight ahead several yards, such as at a rug.
5. Stand with your feet a few inches apart
6. Make sure you can see the toes. (sandals)
7. Start on the healthy side and look down at the toes.
8. Count 1,2,3,4 as you look at the toes
9. Look up at the destination across the room, across at the green carpet, and over at a desk or table.
10. This is your destination for when you begin to walk
11. Jump over to the affected foot, count to 5,6,7,8 as you look at the toes
12. Then look up at the destination again.
13. Then back at to the healthy side, and count to 9,10,11,12

14. Look up at the destination

15. Then back at the affected side and count to 13,14,15,16

16. Take a rest.

This is how marathoners look up from the finish line, straight ahead, to get a look at how far they need to run. They do, this, so they can focus on their target and what they need to do to get there and decide how far they need to go.

That's why you stand in a threshold, as if it is the start of a finish line and so you can get a feel of where you need to go, and start to work this out in your head, but also so the mirror cells know that you have a plan and a purpose for staring down at the toes.

Exercise 9.5: Get ready to walk (use for 2x day)

1. Stand in threshold

2. Look down at the healthy toes, count 1,2,3,4

3. Look over at the affected toes, count 5,6,7,8

4. Look up at your destination across the dining room

5. Point eyes over at the floor cover, such as carpet

6. Look for a few seconds

7. Count out numbers 9,10,11,12 and then push up on the heel of the affected foot.

8. Then push off on the ball of foot on the affected side.

9. Keep walking in a marching band formation

10. Keep counting, 13,14,15,16 as you walk.

11. Walk in a straight line across the room, and as you do keep thinking of the affected foot, and if you can picture how the foot looks in the image.

12. Try to picture how the affected foot and legs look in the image.

13. After the last set of ten steps, pause and take a rest.

14. Take a rest

Showing the brain that you have a reflective image of the feet ahead of time before you start to walk, is a plan, and one that is a purposeful gesture. If you can't form the entire visual image of the affected foot, you are still able to show the brain that you need to step off the feet and use them to walk. This starts to create a permanent memory in the brain of staring at the toes, with the intention of walking.

Walking slowly, as you push off the toes, allows you to study the steps, and work on the parts of the lift-off, that you may still work on. Pushing off the ball of the foot may be a place that you need to study the most because this is often a place when you lose the image.

Practice: looking back as you step off the toes:

1. Stand in threshold

2. Look down at the toes on healthy foot and count 1,2,3,4

3. Then the affected foot and count 5,6,7,8

4. Look up at the destination

5. Lift once off on the healthy foot

6. Take a few steps, slowly

7. Look back at how healthy foot looks, when you push off on the ball of the foot.

8. Do this slowly

9. Then look back at the affected foot, as you push off this foot

10. Do this slowly

11. Take a rest

Do this again four times.

The reason you are looking back at how you lift off on the healthy foot, is so you can see how you use the foot, but also feel how you use the foot. The closer the two feet look when you push off on the foot, the more likely the mirror cells will create a matching image for the feet. This will increase your chances to retain the image of the two feet as you walk and begin to present an image of how some of the legs looks in the image.

Exercise 9.6: Imagine that the affected foot feels and works the same way

1. Stand in threshold

2. Look down at the toes on healthy foot and count 1,2,3,4

3. Then the affected foot and count 5,6,7,8

4. Look up at the destination

5. Lift off once from the healthy foot

6. Take a few steps, slowly

7. Look back at how healthy foot looks, when you push off on the ball of the foot.

8. Notice the tension in the middle of the foot

9. Press off on the ball of the foot

10. Notice the tension in the back of the toes.

11. Do this slowly

12. Then look back at the affected foot, as you push off this foot

13. Do this slowly

14. Try to detect the tension in the middle of the foot

15. Take a rest

Do this again four times.

Lift off slowly, so you can see the exact moves of the feet and feel how the foot feels. This is also a way to notice the differences between how each foot feels, so you know the weaknesses of the affected foot. For example, a weakness might be knowing that you need to lift off the ball of the foot with strength, and you might be lifting off with slightly, less control over this part of the foot. This tells you that you need to work on strengthening the toes, to try and match how you lift off on the other foot.

You may be missing an image of the heel of the foot, and so this might be what is throwing off your walking. This is because the memory for how to lift off the foot, is still weak, and you are getting only some of it back. This image will improve as you get better at trying to make both visual images of the feet look more alike.

Exercise 9.7: Give verbal commands as you step off the toes of the foot (use for 1x day).

1. Stand in threshold
2. Look down at the toes on healthy foot and count 1,2,3,4
3. Then the affected foot and count 5,6,7,8
4. Look up at the destination
5. Lift off once from the healthy foot
6. Take a few steps, slowly
7. Look back at how healthy foot looks, when you push off on the ball of the foot.
8. Notice the tension in the middle of the foot
9. Press off on the ball of the foot
10. Notice the tension in the back of the toes.

11. Do this slowly

12. Then look back at the affected foot, as you push off this foot

13. Do this slowly

14. Say, "this foot looks like the other foot."

15. Take another step, and look back at how to push off the foot

16. Say, "this foot moves like the other foot."

17. Take a rest

Do this again four times.

Saying these prompts tells you that you think that the two feet are alike, even though you may be having some trouble forming an image of the affected one. If you say this and pretend that you believe it, then the mirror cells will think that you are ready to use the foot. They only respond when they hear you say that you think the two motor parts are the same, or that you feel that the motor parts work the same way. This tells the mirror cells that you are planning to use this foot, and that's all they need to hear to know that you are planning an activity with the feet. This will allow them to absorb some of the image, and return some of the motor functions, and then allow you to start to receive some of the memory back for how to visualize how you are moving the foot.

Study the legs in the mirror:

If you have a full-length mirror or one on a bureau that allows you to see the tops of the legs, you can achieve an image of the legs this way. This does involve counting as well, to create that verbal cue you need to attract the mirror cells to your image and be able to show that you are thinking of an activity with the legs.

Exercise 9.8: Stand in front of mirror, and focus on the tops of the legs, to walk (use for 1x day)

1. Stand in front of the mirror

2. Look at the tops of the legs, for up to thirty seconds

3. Keep your eyes on the tops of the legs the whole time

4. After thirty seconds, start walking away from the mirror

5. You will notice that you will know how to walk

6. You will also notice that you are able to form an image of the legs

7. You will also be able to hold onto some of this image

8. You may also notice improved ability to plan and know how long you want to do the task.

Any reflective image that you see in the mirror, is an image that mirror cells can absorb right away. This is because both legs appear identical, and if you are looking at them, then the mirror cells will assume work the same way. They will restore the memory of how the legs work, to you and you will be able to start walking around for about ten to twenty seconds as if you feel that you are alright.

Memories that you get back in the mirror only last for four to ten seconds at a time, after you leave the mirror, and so you will have to keep returning to the mirror to keep using this memory.

Checkpoint:

Do the exercises for four weeks 2x a day. Focus on improving the image of the feet, by looking back at them as you walk, and using verbal prompts to get the attention of mirror cells. The image of the legs will return slowly, in the form of wispy images at first, and then the whole image, after about eight weeks of walking.

References

1. Bentz, John E. M.d. (2015). Can the Brain Heal itself after stroke? Penn Medicine. MyLGHealth.

   http://lghealthhub.org/Brain-Spine-Health/Can-a-brain-heal-itself-after-a-stroke

2. Annabel McDermott, OT; Adam Kagan, B.Sc.; ET. AL. (2019). Mirror Therapy Upper

   Extremity. Canadian Partnership for stroke therapy. Heart and Stroke Foundation.

   https://www.strokengine.ca/en/intervention/mirror-therapy/

3. Perry, Susan. (2013). Neuroanatomy: mirror neurons. *Brainfacts.org.* Retrieved from:
   http://www.brainfacts.org/brain-basics/neuroanatomy/articles/2008/mirror-neurons/

About the Author:

In 2014 I had a stroke. This led to the discovery of the motion memory, and other ways to attract mirror cells. I researched these methods and determined that attracting mirror cells allows motor functions of the brain to return, for a short time. This increases the chances of healing and the ability to use these parts of the brain over time. This method can be used by anyone trying to recover from a stroke or by someone looking to improve their brain functions in general.

www.ingramcontent.com/pod-product-compliance
Lightning Source LLC
Chambersburg PA
CBHW031305280526
45784CB00004B/1998